Eat Well & Feel Great

The Power of Food to Nourish Your Body and Soul

Prutha Desai

©Copyright 2021 Prutha Desai- All rights reserved.

The content contained within this book may not be reproduced, duplicated, or transmitted without direct written permission from the author or the publisher.

Under no circumstances will any blame or legal responsibility be held against the publisher, or author, for any damages, reparation, or monetary loss due to the information contained within this book, either directly or indirectly.

Legal Notice:

This book is copyright protected. It is only for personal use. You cannot amend, distribute, sell, use, quote, or paraphrase any part, or the content within this book, without the consent of the author or publisher.

Disclaimer Notice:

Please note the information contained within this document is for educational and entertainment purposes only. All effort has been executed to present accurate, up-to-date, reliable, complete information. No warranties of any kind are declared or implied. Readers acknowledge that the author is not engaged in the rendering of legal, financial, medical, or professional advice. The content within this book has been derived from various sources. Please consult a licensed professional before attempting any techniques outlined in this book.

By reading this document, the reader agrees that under no circumstances is the author responsible for any losses, direct or indirect, that are incurred as a result of the use of the information contained within this document, including, but not limited to, errors, omissions, or inaccuracies.

ISBN-13: 9798501566095

Contents

Introduction

Have you ever tried to research what diet plan is the healthiest or how to incorporate healthy eating into your routine? If you have, you know that there is a lot of information out there, and some of it can be confusing.

It seems like there are a million different choices when it comes to what diet to follow. Should you follow a low-carb diet or a raw food diet? Should you do a cleanse? Every week there is a new study that highlights the benefit of one diet over another. And there are lots of advertisements for quick fixes. Between the ads and celebrity endorsements, it's hard to know what to believe. And it can be stressful.

The truth is that one diet plan does not fit all because we are not all designed the same way. We all have different health concerns, like high blood pressure, high or low blood sugar, or a family history of heart disease. What may work for one person may not work for another. And quick-fix diets are just that. They are quick fixes, meant to take some weight off quickly. But they aren't sustainable or healthy.

And much of what we eat these days can't be classified as real food. There's a prevalence of processed, convenience food that contains ingredients that most of us can't pronounce. In fact, more than half of Americans' calories come from "ultra-processed foods," according to a 2016 study (Beck, 2016).

Every time you walk into a grocery store, you are bombarded with choices, and most of them don't seem that great. There are entire aisles for chips, pop, and chocolate bars. And never mind the cookie aisle. Not to say that you should never eat these things as an occasional treat. But it's getting trickier to figure out how to choose foods that nourish us when there are convenient, tasty temptations all around.

If you're reading this book, you are probably interested in learning more about healthy eating and what that looks like for you. You have probably made a decision not to eat junky, processed foods any longer and want to learn how to make better choices for your body.

This book is not about the latest diet or any quick fixes. It's about a lifestyle and a way to approach what and how you eat. You will learn the importance of real, unprocessed food and how to eat mindfully. You will also learn simple, sustainable habits that will bring you joy.

As you read through the chapters, you'll become knowledgeable about how to shop for and incorporate healthy, real food into your daily meal planning. You'll learn how whole foods nourish and help heal your body. And you'll see how eating real food can have a positive impact on your overall health and well-being. You will know how to change your habits so that healthy eating becomes second nature.

Eating real whole foods is about changing your lifestyle. It's not about embracing a quick fix. It means letting go of processed, unhealthy foods that do not provide your body any nutritional value. It's about incorporating more vegetables, lean proteins, healthy fats, and unrefined grains into more of your meals.

You have so many decisions to make in your daily life. What to eat should be one of the easier decisions. It should bring you joy and not be stressful. Once you have finished this book, you will know how to change your habits so that eating healthy foods becomes automatic for you. You will also understand that real food has the power to restore and heal your body and mind if you let it.

Here's to eating healthy and to a happy and healthy life!

Chapter 1: Eat Well for Life

What are some of your fondest memories? They probably involve sitting with family or friends, enjoying delicious and wholesome food. Maybe you remember how much better a bowl of homemade chicken noodle soup made you feel when you last had a cold. Or how a good piece of dark chocolate took the edge off a stressful day. Food is so much more than just fuel to live. It nourishes us, heals us, and brings us together with family and friends.

Why We Eat

The reason we eat is simple: We need food to live. Just like our electronic devices need to be plugged in to be charged, we need food, so we stay charged to do the things we need and want to do.

Our bodies are made up of cells. These cells help perform our body's tasks. Some examples of actions the cells are responsible for are making hormones, growing muscles, producing energy, and building bones.

The cells in your body need proper nutrition so they can function properly. But how do the cells get their nutrients, you might be wondering. The answer is your digestive system releases nutrients from the food you eat.

Your digestive system breaks down the nutrients into the form of glucose. Once the nutrients are released, your cells use the glucose to do their jobs, whether that's building muscles or sustaining your breathing.

Without proper food and nutrition, your cells would not be able to perform their tasks properly.

The way we get our food has changed over time. One of the biggest changes over the last 50 years is how industrialized food production has become. Another major change is the prevalence of fast-food chains.

People are eating more sugar than they used to. Part of this is because the sugar industry pays for research that minimizes the negative effects and risks of sugar to peoples' health (Domonoske, 2019). Yearly consumption of sugar has risen to 152 pounds per person from 123 pounds in 1970 (Leake, 2013).

And people aren't just eating sugar to get that sweetness in their diet. High-fructose corn syrup is in many processed items that are on the grocery shelves, including soda.

To be fair, highly processed food can be addictive. In February 2021, Ashley Gearhardt, associate professor in the psychology department at the University of Michigan, compared processed foods, including fries, frozen pizza, potato chips, and packaged cookies, to addictive drugs (Gearhardt & Hebebrand, 2021). This means people who are addicted to processed foods experience intense cravings, an inability to cut back on eating these foods even if they experience negative consequences, and a loss of control.

Processed food is addictive because it provides pleasure. It is stripped of its natural state, including the removal of protein, fiber, and water, which slow the absorption of the food. Then the ingredients that bring the most pleasure are refined so that they are easily and quickly absorbed into the bloodstream. This highlights the areas of the brain that are in charge of motivation and reward (O'Connor, 2021). The more reward you get, the more motivated you are to get more of the reward.

On the opposite end of the spectrum from processed food is real food. Unprocessed food gives your body the minerals and vitamins it needs to function properly. For example, one cup of broccoli has more than 100 percent of the recommended daily intake for vitamin C. Real food also provides nutrients and antioxidants, like magnesium and healthy fats, that keep your heart healthy.

Real food is also naturally lower in sugar than processed food which helps protect your body from obesity, diabetes, liver, and heart disease. It is also higher in fiber which helps your digestive system function properly.

It's Okay to Be Confused and Frustrated

If you look online for current nutrition and diet information, you know that there is a lot of information and misinformation. There are articles and entire websites dedicated to diets like vegan, paleo, keto, macros, and intermittent fasting. You'll see the pros and cons of each diet, how many calories you need in a day, what types of food you should and should not eat and how much you should exercise. It can be completely overwhelming.

There is also lots of conflicting information about what foods to avoid. It seems like every week, there is a new study that touts the benefits of a certain food, only to be refuted the following week by a new study that shows how bad that food is.

There is also misinformation out there about how healthy eating means you have to eat bland, flavorless food. You may have also heard that if you eat healthily, you must never eat treats again.

It is okay to be confused and frustrated by all of the information! With all of the advice out there, it is hard to know where to begin and what to eat.

But don't throw in the towel yet. Because the answer is by taking small steps, one day at a time, you can learn how to incorporate real, whole foods into your routine. You'll see that the results will speak for themselves.

Eat Better, Feel Better, Do Better

Food has the power to nourish and heal us. By eating whole foods, you will see real changes not only in your appearance but in your mood and energy levels. There is no question that by eating a diet rich in real foods, you will feel like the best version of yourself. I encourage you to read on to learn more about the steps you can take to make whole foods part of your daily diet. And once you get on that whole food kick, you'll want to continue to eat better because you'll feel better and do better.

Chapter 2: Food Groups Explained

You may have seen different versions of the basic food groups as you were growing up. Below, you'll find information on the foods that your body needs to function properly so that you can live your best life.

Protein

Protein is important because it gives you the energy to do all of the things that you want to do. You need protein to build, maintain, repair cells, organs, and tissues in your body. Other benefits of protein are it helps you think clearly, it can help with your response to stress, depression, and anxiety, and it can help you maintain a healthy weight by making you feel full for longer. Protein also helps give you healthy skin, nails, and hair.

Protein is made up of organic compounds called amino acids. When your system digests protein, the amino acids are left. There are essential and non-essential amino acids. Our bodies can't produce the essential amino acids, so it is necessary for us to get our essential amino acids from food. On the flip side, our bodies can make non-essential amino acids, so it isn't necessary to get them from food.

There is high-quality and low-quality protein. The quality is determined by the amount of essential amino acids in the food item. Sources of complete protein usually come from animal products like meat, eggs, poultry, dairy, and fish. If you're a vegetarian or vegan, the most complete source of plant-based protein is soybeans. Other good plant-based sources of protein are whole grains, legumes, nuts, and seeds.

Examples of healthy sources of protein are nuts and seeds (which also have fiber and good fats), soy products like tofu (which are high in protein and low-fat), beans (they also contain fiber), dairy products like yogurt and cheese, lean poultry, and fish. Look for unsalted nuts and low-sodium beans so that you're not increasing your salt intake when you eat these foods.

Not all protein is good for you, though. For example, things like processed lunch meats may contain protein; however, they also have too much salt, which can lead to health problems like high blood pressure.

Some simple ways you can incorporate more healthy protein into your diet include snacking on nuts instead of potato chips, replacing your dessert with some yogurt, and ditching a pizza for some grilled fish.

If you do not consume meat, for whatever reason, there are other healthy options. Soy products are high in protein. For example, half a cup of firm tofu contains around 10 grams of protein. Half a cup of edamame beans, which are immature soybeans, contains 8.5 grams of protein. And tempeh, made from fermented soybeans, has 15 grams of protein.

Use tofu in stir-fries or in soup. Steam edamame, then munch on it, out of the pod or shell edamame, and add it to your pasta sauce. You can marinate or bake tempeh and enjoy it in a sandwich or stir fry.

Other non-meat sources of protein include lentils, chickpeas, almonds, peanuts, spirulina, quinoa, hemp and chia seeds, and seitan.

Adults need about 0.8 grams of protein per kilogram of body weight (Pendick, 2015). Examples of the amount of protein you can get in certain foods include 3 ounces of skinless chicken: 28 grams of protein; 3 ounces of salmon: 22 grams of protein; half-cup of pinto beans: 11 grams of protein; 1 ounce of soy nuts: 12 grams of protein; 6 ounces of Greek yogurt: 18 grams of protein (Petre, 2019).

Carbohydrates

You have probably read a lot of information about carbohydrates or carbs. Carbs have been vilified over the years because there are lots of bad carbs out there. But the truth is that our bodies need some carbs. And no, not in the form of chips!

If you are wondering what exactly carbs are, look no further. Carbs are starches, fibers, and sugars found in milk products, vegetables, fruits, and grains. They are considered macronutrients which means that they are one of the ways our body gets energy or calories.

Our bodies turn carbs into sugar, like fructose and glucose, during digestion. Our small intestine absorbs the sugars. The sugars then enter our bloodstream and go to our liver. Our liver then changes the sugar into glucose which also goes into our bloodstream. The glucose travels with insulin, and it is then changed into fuel for our bodies so that we can do the things we need and want to do.

Glucose is also important to the healthy function of our brains because it can't use other sources of fuel, such as fat or protein, for energy (Selhub, 2018). Carbs influence our mood, and memory and studies have linked our social decision-making skills and carbs (Strang et al., 2017).

Some studies suggest that including a healthy level of carbs in our diet can help our mental health. One study found that people on low-carb diets had more anger, depression, and anxiety than people that consumed normal or higher levels of carbs (Brinkworth et al., 2009).

If you don't get enough carbs in your diet, it could be problematic. Carbs provide fuel for your body. Without fuel, you will have no energy. Also, without the glucose your body uses from the carbs, your central nervous system can be distressed, leading to you feeling dizzy or having a mental and physical weakness.

If your body doesn't have enough carbs stored, it will use protein for fuel. The problem with that is your body needs protein to make muscles. If your body uses protein instead of carbs for fuel, your kidneys will suffer. This could lead to your body passing painful byproducts in your urine.

If you don't eat enough carbs, you may not get enough fiber which could then lead to constipation and problems with your digestive system.

You probably have heard that there are two types of carbs: simple and complex. What makes these types of carbs different is their chemical structure and how quickly our system absorbs and digests the sugar in carbs.

Our bodies digest and absorb simple carbs quicker and more easily than complex carbs. Simple carbs have one or two sugars and galactose, which is found in milk products. Simple carbs include table sugar, some fruit juices, candy, syrups, soda, and honey. These products are full of empty calories.

Complex carbs contain three or more sugars. They are often starchy and can be found in grain products like crackers, pasta, rice, and bread. Some vegetables are high in starch, like corn, sweet and white potatoes, and butternut squash. It is best to try to get mostly complex carbs in your diet.

What we consider 'good' carbs are carbs that are moderate to low in calories. They are high in nutrients, don't have refined sugars and grains, and high in naturally occurring fiber. These carbs are also low in sodium and saturated fat and have very low to zero cholesterol and trans fats.

Good carbs include whole grain foods like brown rice, whole wheat pasta, and whole grain bread. These foods contain fiber, which is important because it helps your digestive system function properly and it helps regulate your blood sugar levels. Foods with fiber take longer to be digested, which means the glucose in these foods goes into your bloodstream slowly. Whole grain foods also contain nutrients your body needs, like B vitamins, vitamin E, and magnesium.

Some foods that are considered 'superfoods' because of their high levels of nutrients contain carbs. Think of sweet potatoes, leafy greens, berries, and apples.

On the opposite end are the bad carbs. These carbs are high in empty calories. They contain lots of refined sugar, like white sugar and corn syrup. They also have lots of refined grains, like white flour, they contain little to no nutrients, and they are low in fiber. Bad carbs are high in sodium, and they sometimes contain high levels of trans fats, cholesterol, and saturated fat.

These types of carbs include white rice, white pasta, donuts, cookies, and cakes. These foods have had their fiber and nutrients removed so the glucose in them can get into your bloodstream faster, raising your blood sugar levels.

Keeping your blood sugar levels consistent is important not only because it can help prevent type 2 diabetes but also it helps regulate your mood. Think of when you eat something sweet, like a donut. You probably feel elated while you're eating it. But shortly afterward, you likely feel sleepy and maybe a bit cranky, which is a result of the blood-sugar spike and crash.

This is because the sugar from the donut quickly went into your bloodstream. That's when you feel energized. But the spike in blood sugar causes your body to produce more insulin to try and balance your blood sugar levels. And that is when you crash. Avoid blood sugar spikes and crashes by avoiding unhealthy carbs.

Some tips for avoiding unhealthy carbs include choosing whole grains, like brown rice and whole wheat bread. When you're grocery shopping, make sure you look at the ingredient list to see that it says "100% whole grain." Avoid things like cake, cookies, and donuts because they contain refined sugars.

You might want to try adding barley into your diet. You can use it in soup instead of rice or pasta. Substitute brown rice for white rice in your recipes. And try making a stir fry with quinoa.

Vegetables

As a kid, you were probably told to eat your vegetables. And being a kid, you probably asked why. Maybe you got the typical, "Because I said so." Or maybe you were told that you should eat your vegetables because they are good for you, but you weren't told how they are good for you.

Vegetables contain many nutrients, including potassium. Potassium helps maintain healthy blood pressure. You can find potassium in sweet potatoes, white beans, tomatoes, lima beans, spinach, lentils, soybeans, and beet greens.

You can also find fiber in vegetables. As you read earlier, fiber is important in maintaining a healthy digestive system. Fiber helps keep your cholesterol in check and may also reduce your risk of heart disease.

Vegetables contain vitamin A and C. Vitamin A helps protect against infections. It also helps keep your skin and eyes healthy.

Vitamin C helps your body absorb iron. It keeps your gums and teeth healthy, and it helps heal cuts.

Eating vegetables can reduce your chance of getting heart disease, and it reduces your chance of having a stroke or heart attack. If you eat your vegetables, you might also be protected against certain types of cancer.

If you're wondering about specific vegetables and their nutritional content, you'll find more information about some popular vegetables below.

One of the healthiest vegetables is spinach. Spinach contains iron, antioxidants, and calcium. If you don't eat meat or dairy, spinach is a good substitute because of its high calcium and iron content. It also contains vitamin K, which is essential for healthy, strong bones because it improves the absorption of calcium.

One common vegetable that packs a nutritional punch is broccoli. Broccoli is a cruciferous vegetable in the same family as kale, cauliflower, and cabbage. Broccoli has vitamin K and vitamin C. You can cook broccoli in many different ways, including roasting or steaming it and blending it with soup.

Kale is another common, popular vegetable that is packed with nutrients. Kale contains vitamins A, K, and C. Research shows that kale juice can help reduce blood sugar levels, along with blood pressure and blood cholesterol (Han et al., 2015). If you haven't tried kale and are unsure how to eat it, you can try steaming it and eating it with pasta or putting it on a sandwich. You can also try making kale chips, but more on that later!

Carrots are a popular vegetable because they are tasty, crunchy, and versatile. Eat them as a snack, as a side dish, or as a salad topping! Carrots contain vitamin A, which is in the form of beta carotene. Vitamin A is important for healthy eyesight.

Sweet potatoes are another superior vegetable. This is because they have vitamins A, B6, C, potassium, and beta carotene, a pigment that may help improve eye health. Sweet potatoes are low on the glycemic index and are rich in fiber, making them a great choice for people with diabetes.

Tomatoes are actually a fruit, but most people eat them in savory dishes like they do with other vegetables. Tomatoes contain potassium and vitamin C. They also have lycopene, which is an antioxidant that may help prevent certain types of cancers. They also contain zeaxanthin and lutein, both of which may protect vision.

Another type of fruit that we normally treat as a vegetable is a bell pepper. Bell peppers come in different colors, ranging from green to red. The colors represent the different states of ripeness. Peppers contain fiber, vitamins B6 and C, folate, potassium, and manganese.

If you like sauerkraut from cabbage or pickles from cucumber, you are in luck! Not only do fermented vegetables contain all of the nutrients as their unfermented peer, but they also provide your body with probiotics. Probiotics are the beneficial bacteria that naturally live in your body. Eating foods with probiotics can improve your gut health.

It is recommended that adults eat between two to four cups of vegetables per day. This might sound like a lot, but you'd be surprised at how fast you can get your daily recommended intake. It could look like:

- one large bell pepper (equals one cup) in your lunch and dinner salad
- two medium carrots (equals one cup) in your lunch and dinner salad or chopped up as a crunchy snack with some hummus as a dip
- one large tomato (equals one cup) in your lunch and dinner salad
- one avocado (equals one cup), on toast or in a salad
- two cups of raw salad greens (equals one cup) in your lunch and dinner salad

If you do not currently eat the daily recommended intake of vegetables, start slowly. Try making avocado toast for lunch and having a big side salad at dinner. The important thing is that you start. Because it's important to eat your vegetables!

Fruits

Fruits are a food group that is naturally delicious and nutritious. They are naturally cholesterol-free. Many fruits are also low in fat, calories, and sodium.

If you're wondering what is included in the fruit food group, the answer is all fruit and 100 percent fruit juice. You can eat your fruits fresh, frozen, canned, or dried. They can be pureed or cooked. And half of your daily fruit should come from actual fruit instead of 100 percent fruit juice.

Many fruits contain potassium. As you read earlier, potassium helps maintain healthy blood pressure. You can find potassium in prunes, bananas, dried peaches, cantaloupe, guava, kiwi, and orange juice.

Fruits also contain fiber which, as you now know, is important in keeping your digestive system healthy. It also helps reduce cholesterol levels and can help reduce the risk of heart disease. The best way to get your fiber is by eating fruits, as fruit juices have very little fiber.

Like vegetables, fruits also contain vitamin C, which keeps gums and teeth healthy, helps your body absorb iron, contributes to the growth and repair of body tissues, and helps heal cuts.

Wondering about specific fruits and their nutritional content? See information about some popular fruits below.

Lemons are a popular citrus fruit that, like other citrus fruits, have vitamins A, B6, and C and antioxidants. The antioxidants clean up free radicals in our bodies that can lead to cancer. Lemons also contain folic acid, pectin, and potassium. The juice of one lemon has 49 milligrams of potassium, 18.6 milligrams of vitamin C, and 3 milligrams of calcium. You can squeeze lemon over fish or add it to a glass of water as a natural flavor.

Oranges are another citrus fruit that packs a nutritional punch. They have the highest level of vitamin C. One medium orange contains 117 percent of a person's recommended daily intake of vitamin C (National Institutes of Health, 2016). Vitamin C is an antioxidant that is important for a healthy immune system. The reason for this is that vitamin C helps the body absorb iron from plant-based food. Since our bodies can't make vitamin C, it is important that we get it from our food. One 141-gram orange has 3.4 grams of fiber, 61 milligrams of calcium, 14 milligrams of magnesium, 238 milligrams of potassium, and 63.5 milligrams of vitamin C. You can enjoy an orange as it is or drink orange juice.

Strawberries are a delicious, juicy fruit. Strawberry seeds contain high levels of fiber. They also contain vitamins A and B6. Strawberries also have flavonoids that have anti-inflammatory properties and may help heart health. Three large strawberries have 1.1 grams of fiber, 9 milligrams of calcium, 7 milligrams of magnesium, 31.8 milligrams of vitamin C, and 83 milligrams of potassium. You can enjoy strawberries just as they are, chopped up over a salad, over your cereal, or in a smoothie.

Grapefruits come in pink, white, and red varieties, and they are chock-full of minerals and vitamins. Half a grapefruit has 2 grams of fiber, 27 grams of calcium, 11 grams of magnesium, 166 grams of potassium, and 38.4 grams of vitamin C. Grapefruits also contain flavonoids that can help protect against inflammation and cancer. Enjoy a grapefruit as part of your breakfast, or squeeze grapefruit juice in a glass to enjoy it as a beverage.

Blackberries are another popular fruit that can keep you in good health. Like strawberries, the seeds in blackberries contain high amounts of fiber which helps with heart and gut health. Half a cup of blackberries has 3.8 grams of fiber, 21 milligrams of calcium, 14 milligrams of magnesium, 117 milligrams of potassium, and 15.1 milligrams of vitamin C. Top your breakfast cereal with blackberries, add them to some yogurt or make them part of your smoothie.

Blueberries are considered a superfood because of their nutritional qualities. They have anthocyanin, an antioxidant that can help protect against stroke, cancers, and heart disease. Half a cup of blueberries contains 1.8 grams of fiber, 4 milligrams of calcium, 57 milligrams of potassium, and 7.2 milligrams of vitamin C.

You've probably heard the saying, "an apple a day keeps the doctor away." Apples are easy to pack in your lunch, and they provide a satisfying crunch. They contain high amounts of fiber and pectin, which means they are excellent for your heart and your gut. One medium apple contains 4.4 grams of fiber, 195 milligrams of potassium, 11 milligrams of calcium, and 8.4 milligrams of vitamin C. Eat apples whole or cut them up and top with peanut butter.

Bananas are a very popular fruit that comes in their own packaging, making them very convenient to pack as part of a lunch or a snack. Bananas are a great source of energy. One banana has about 105 calories and 26.95 carbs. They are also high in fiber. One medium banana has 6 milligrams of calcium, 32 milligrams of magnesium, and 10.3 milligrams of vitamin C. Eat a banana on its own, slice it and put it on top of waffles or pancakes, or add it to a smoothie.

Avocados contain oleic acid, a monounsaturated fat, which is known to help lower cholesterol levels. According to the American Health Association, eating healthy fats to maintain cholesterol levels can reduce the risk of stroke and heart disease. Avocados also contain potassium and lutein. Half an avocado has 2.01 grams of protein, 6.7 grams of fiber, 12 milligrams of calcium, 29 milligrams of magnesium, 487 milligrams of potassium, and 10.1 milligrams of vitamin C.

It's recommended that adults eat between one and a half cups to two and a half cups of fruit per day. This could look like this:

- half a large apple or one small apple (equals one cup)
- one cup of applesauce
- one large banana (equals one cup)
- one large orange (equals one cup)

If you do not currently eat the suggested daily servings of fruit, start slowly. Try having a banana as an afternoon snack or cut up an apple and enjoy it as a crunchy snack while you are watching TV.

Dairy

Dairy foods contain nutrients and fats that help build strong bones. This is because dairy has vitamin D, calcium, and phosphorus which are all important for your bones. Dairy also has potassium.

Fermented dairy foods, like yogurt, contain healthy gut bacteria, which can help with your digestive health.

If you are lactose intolerant, there are lactose-free options that you can buy. These products contain the same amount of vitamin D and calcium as regular dairy products.

If you're wondering how many nutrients are in one cup of milk (237 ml), it contains the following percentages of your daily recommended intake: 28 percent of calcium, 24 percent of vitamin D, 18 percent of vitamin B12, and 10 percent of potassium.

Yogurt is a popular dairy product made from fermenting milk with yogurt culture. It can be enjoyed as a snack, as part of breakfast, or in a smoothie. Unsweetened, natural yogurt offers the most health benefits.

Natural yogurt, without any sweeteners, is high in calcium and B vitamins. One cup of natural yogurt contains 49 percent of an adult's calcium needs (Elliott, 2017). Natural yogurt is also high in phosphorus, magnesium, and potassium, which help in regulating blood pressure and improving bone health. Yogurt is also high in protein. And some varieties of yogurt, like yogurts that contain live, active cultures, can help with gut health.

Look for grass-fed dairy products as these have more omega-3 fatty acids and are generally considered healthier because they're higher in fat-soluble vitamins like vitamin K2, which helps regulate calcium metabolism. It also supports bone and heart health.

Dairy Substitutes

If you cannot or will not consume dairy products, for whatever reason, there are other healthy options.

One of the most popular alternatives to dairy milk is soy milk. Soy milk has been used in certain cultures for a long time. It is made by extracting the liquid from soybeans. You can buy soy milk unsweetened, sweetened, and flavored. You can also find soy milk that has been fortified with vitamins A and D and calcium. One cup of plain soy milk provides 6.34 grams of protein, 2.68 micrograms of vitamin D, 2.07 micrograms of vitamin B 12, 300 milligrams of calcium, 298 milligrams of potassium, and 0.488 grams of fiber. Soy milk also contains isoflavones, naturally occurring antioxidants, which are associated with a lowered risk of heart disease. Look for unsweetened, organic or non-genetically modified soy milk.

Coconut milk makes an excellent dairy milk substitute because it has a texture that is closest to that of dairy milk. If you have food allergies, coconut milk can make a great alternative because it is naturally gluten and soy-free. Coconut milk is made using the white flesh inside a coconut. Coconuts have lauric acid, which may support a healthy immune system. One cup of canned, raw coconut milk contains 4.57 grams of protein, 41 milligrams of calcium, 497 milligrams of potassium, 104 milligrams of magnesium, 7.46 milligrams of iron, and 2.30 milligrams of vitamin C.

Another good substitute for dairy milk for people with allergies is rice milk. Rice milk is usually free from nuts, gluten, and soy. It is made from boiled rice, brown rice starch, and brown rice syrup. Rice milk is quite low in protein when compared to dairy or soy milk. It also has less calcium than dairy milk so if you want something with more dairy, look for calcium-fortified rice milk.

Almond milk is another popular dairy milk substitute. It is made from ground almonds and water. It is also sometimes fortified with minerals and vitamins, but it has less protein than soy or dairy milk, so if you are looking for a non-dairy alternative with more protein, it is best to consume soy milk.

There are other alternatives to dairy milk, and they include flax, oat, potato, quinoa, sunflower, and hemp milk.

Grains, Legumes, Beans

Whole grains can be considered a nutritional powerhouse. This is because they have three parts: the germ, endosperm, and the bran. Each of these parts contains nutrients.

The germ is the seed core where growth happens. It has healthy fats, B vitamins, vitamin E, and antioxidants. The endosperm is the layer on the very inside, and it has carbohydrates, protein, and some minerals and B vitamins. Finally, the bran, which is the outer layer, is rich in fiber and provides you with B vitamins, copper, zinc, iron, antioxidants, and magnesium ("Whole Grains", 2018).

Now, let's look at the nutrition of whole grains. Fiber and bran slow glucose from breaking down into starch. This helps keep your blood sugar steady and prevents blood sugar spikes. You now know the health benefits of fiber and how it is good for your digestive system, and that it helps control cholesterol levels. Fiber may also be helpful in preventing small blood clots that can lead to strokes and heart attacks. Minerals like selenium, magnesium, and copper, which are all found in whole grains, may protect you against certain types of cancer.

It's recommended that adults eat six ounces of grain foods daily, based on a 2000-calorie diet. The majority of this should come from whole grains because of their superior nutritional value over refined grains. When shopping for grain products, check the ingredient list to make sure that 100 percent of whole grains are listed as the first or second ingredient.

The best way to consume whole grains is to make sure they're unprocessed. Unprocessed whole grains include amaranth, barley, spelt, millet, quinoa, wild rice, oats, rye, bulgur, brown rice, and buckwheat.

Legumes are plants that have leaves, stems, seeds, and pods. They include chickpeas, black beans, and peanuts. Legumes don't contain a lot of saturated fat. They are also a great source of plant protein. Half a cup of cooked beans contains between six and nine grams of protein. Legumes' protein content and low levels of saturated fat make them an excellent substitute for red meat.

Legumes are packed with nutrients, like calcium, potassium, B vitamins, zinc, and antioxidants. They also contain fiber.

If you're curious how much nutrition is packed in certain legumes, three ounces of black beans contains 7.5 grams of fiber, 7.6 grams of protein, 23 milligrams of calcium, 1.8 milligrams of iron, and 305 milligrams of potassium.

If you're wondering how you can add more legumes to your diet, you can try adding chickpeas or another type of bean to soup or pasta. You can add them whole or blend them for a creamier texture. You can cook legumes from their dried versions or use canned or frozen legumes. Instead of eating a sandwich with processed meats, try having a peanut butter sandwich.

Pulses are the edible seeds from a legume plant. They include beans, lentils, and peas. To help make the distinction, a pea pod is a legume because it's the actual plant, but the pea is the seed inside and is a pulse.

Beans have amino acids, the protein your body uses to make and heal tissues, like muscle, bone, hair, skin, and blood. As with legumes, you can use dried, canned, or frozen beans in your cooking. Bean varieties include black beans, soybeans, garbanzo beans, pinto beans, and red beans.

Along with protein, beans also contain folate, which helps make healthy red blood cells. Beans also contain antioxidants that protect your body from free radicals, damaging chemicals that can cause cell damage and disease.

Getting more beans in your diet can be simple. Try making a black bean burrito bowl with brown rice. Top with avocado, tomato, and cilantro for a tasty lunch or dinner. You can sprinkle beans on a salad or use hummus as a spread on a sandwich. Try adding pureed black beans as a flour substitute in brownies for a rich dessert.

Fats

You've probably read that fat isn't good for you, especially if you've researched certain diets. But the truth is that your body needs certain types of fat because fat is an energy source. It also helps your body absorb minerals and vitamins. Fat is important for muscle movement, blood clotting, and preventing inflammation. Your body uses fat to build cell membranes and the sheaths surrounding your nerves.

Not all fats are the same. Incorporate good fats, like polyunsaturated and monounsaturated, to reap the benefits for your long-term health. These good fats come from vegetables, seeds, fish, and nuts. Good fats are liquid at room temperature.

You'll find polyunsaturated fats in sunflower oil, corn oil, and safflower oil. You actually need polyunsaturated fats, but your body can't make them. Your body uses these fats to build the covering of nerves and your cell membranes. Polyunsaturated fats also help with blood clotting, inflammation, and muscle movement.

Omega-3 fatty acids and omega-6 fatty acids are the two types of polyunsaturated fats. Omega-3 fatty acids have many benefits, including potentially preventing heart disease and stroke, reducing blood pressure, and lowering triglycerides. You can find omega-3 fatty acids in flaxseeds, canola oil, walnuts, and fatty fish like mackerel, salmon, and sardines.

Omega-6 fatty acids may protect against heart disease also. You can find these fats in oils like walnut, soybean, and safflower.

The fat you want to stay away from is trans fat. Trans fat is a byproduct of hydrogenation which turns healthy oils into solids. This prevents them from going rancid. There are no health benefits to eating trans fats, and these fats have been officially banned in the United States and other countries.

Eating foods that contain trans fats increases harmful cholesterol in your system and reduces the amount of beneficial cholesterol (yes! there is beneficial cholesterol). Trans fats also create inflammation in your body, which can cause diabetes, stroke, and heart disease. Trans fats can also increase your risk of getting type 2 because they contribute to insulin resistance.

Trans fat increases harmful cholesterol in your system, which then can cause your arteries to clog. It's best to stick with the good fats!

Chapter 3: Food Is Medicine

Eating real food makes us less hungry and keeps our bodies healthy. But it can also prevent and partially treat certain ailments in our bodies.

Chronic Disease

Inflammation in the body can cause issues with your immune system that lead to chronic diseases. Inflammation happens when your body realizes there is something foreign, for example, plant pollen or a chemical. Short periods of inflammation protect your health, but sometimes inflammation can last longer-term. And ongoing inflammation can lead to heart disease, cancer, arthritis, diabetes, Alzheimer's, and depression.

There are certain foods that can cause inflammation in your body, and you probably won't be surprised when you see what they are. Things like fried foods, shortening or margarine, and refined carbs can all cause inflammation. It is best to try and avoid these foods if you can. But you already know that now!

One of the best ways to control inflammation is with your diet. Some of the best anti-inflammatory foods are green leafy vegetables, nuts, olive oil, fatty fish, tomatoes, and fruits like blueberries, oranges, cherries, and strawberries. These foods are high in antioxidants, and the fruits and vegetables contain protective compounds that reduce inflammation.

Many whole foods can help reduce your chances of getting a chronic disease, like heart disease. A diet rich in vegetables, fruits, quality dairy products, protein, and whole grains can help keep your heart healthy, reducing your chances of getting heart disease. While trans fat and salt are linked to an increased chance of heart disease.

You read in chapter 2 about the health benefits of grains. An Iowa Women's Health Study showed a connection between eating whole grains and a lower death rate from inflammatory and infection causes, including gout, asthma, rheumatoid arthritis, Crohn's disease, and ulcerative colitis (Jacobs et al., 2007). The study went on to say that compared to women who never or rarely ate whole grain foods, women who ate at least two servings a day had a 30 percent less chance of dying from an inflammation-related condition.

Eating at least two servings a day of whole grains instead of refined grains can help reduce the risk of getting type 2 diabetes. The components of whole grains slow the absorption of food and help prevent spikes in blood sugar, unlike refined grains that usually have a higher glycemic load and fewer nutrients and fiber.

Beans have many positive effects on your health. Eating beans on a regular basis can also lessen the chance of dying from a heart attack or of having other heart issues (Marventano et al., 2016). And some research shows that the nutrients in beans might help lower cholesterol which contributes to heart disease (Bell et al., 2018). Beans can also help stabilize blood sugar levels and might reduce the risk of getting type 2 diabetes.

As you read in chapter 2, you know that fruits and vegetables are good for you, and they can reduce your chance of heart disease and stroke. A 2014 study showed that participants who ate more fruits and vegetables reduced their risk of death from cardiovascular disease. The average reduction in risk was four percent for each additional serving of fruits and vegetables per day (Harvard School of Public Health, 2018).

One group of vegetables, known as cruciferous, have been studied for their cancer-preventing properties. Some examples of cruciferous vegetables are broccoli, bok choy, rutabaga, cauliflower, Brussels sprouts, cabbage, kale, and radishes. The most popular and most consumed cruciferous vegetable in the United States is broccoli.

Cruciferous vegetables have many nutrients, including vitamins K, E, and C, beta-carotene, and lutein. And they are high in fiber. These vegetables also contain something called glucosinolates, chemicals that contain sulfur which give cruciferous vegetables their unique smell and bitter flavor.

Without getting too technical, when you prepare, chew, and digest cruciferous vegetables, the glucosinolates break down to form compounds that have been studied for their effects on preventing cancer.

Research has shown that some of these compounds impede cancer development in certain organs in mice and rats, including the stomach, breast, colon, lung, liver, and bladder ("Cruciferous Vegetables and Cancer Prevention", 2010).

The studies indicate the compounds in cruciferous vegetables protect against cancer by helping to inactivate carcinogens. The compounds are also anti-inflammatory, antibacterial, and impede tumor blood vessel formation.

Some research indicates that tomatoes may help protect men from prostate cancer. Lycopene, a pigment that makes tomatoes red, might be the reason (Harvard School of Public Health, 2018). Similar studies suggest that eating tomatoes, cooked tomato products, and other bright fruits and vegetables may reduce the risk of mouth, lung, and throat cancer.

Mental Health

Usually, when you think of eating a healthy diet, it is because you want to take charge of your physical health. But your diet affects your mental health as well.

Your brain does a lot. It does your thinking. It takes care of your senses, your breathing, and your movements. It works while you're awake and while you're asleep. And it needs some sort of fuel to keep it functioning like the well-oiled machine that it is.

Eating a diet rich in whole foods helps nourish your brain because the antioxidants, minerals, and vitamins protect it from oxidative stress, which is the free radicals, or waste, made when your body uses oxygen. These free radicals can cause cell damage.

A diet high in refined sugar can hurt your brain. The sugar spikes you get from eating foods with refined sugars hurt your body's ability to regulate insulin, and they also cause oxidative stress and inflammation in your brain. Studies have shown a connection between impaired brain function and a diet high in refined sugars (Selhub, 2018). A diet high in refined sugars can also worsen mood disorders like depression.

You've probably heard about serotonin, the "feel-good" hormone that is found in some foods. Serotonin is actually a neurotransmitter. It helps impede pain and regulates mood, sleep, and appetite.

A million nerve cells, or neurons, line your gastrointestinal tract. This is where around 95% of serotonin is produced in your body. And the amount of "good bacteria" in your intestinal microbiome influences the neurons and the production of serotonin (Selhub, 2018). So if you think about it, it makes sense that you would want to keep your digestive system healthy because it affects your mood and emotions.

The good bacteria found in probiotic foods like yogurt and sauerkraut are important to your health. They make a barrier between toxins and your body by protecting the lining of your intestines. They also help you absorb nutrients from your food.

Studies show that people who eat diets rich in fruits, vegetables, fish, seafood, and unprocessed grains have a 25 to 35 percent lower chance of getting depression than those who eat processed foods and sugar. The people in the study also ate fermented foods, which, as you know, are natural probiotics.

Try to notice how different foods make you feel as you are eating them and the day after. If something doesn't feel right physically, or you feel that you're in a fog or feeling down, maybe try removing some of the foods you have been eating and replace them with a healthier alternative.

Real Food Properties

As you've read above, not all food is the same. If you are still wondering what real food is, it is food that you can eat while it's in its most natural form. It hasn't been modified from its original version. It hasn't been processed, refined, or had sugar, salt, dyes, fats, or preservatives added to it.

Food that is free of preservatives and that will spoil sooner rather than later is an example of real food. Usually, you can find real food on the outer edges of your grocery store and not in the inner aisles.

Real food includes fresh vegetables and fruit, unsalted seeds and nuts, whole grains, dairy products, legumes and beans, and lean proteins.

By contrast, processed foods have been engineered. They have sugar, salt, and chemical preservatives added to them. Processed foods are typically mass-produced, contain specialized ingredients (including saturated and trans fats), and have a long freezer or shelf life. They come in a jar or box. Processed food has very little or no fiber, very little omega-3 fatty acids, too much salt, and too many trans fats.

Processed foods include potato chips, cookies, bottled salad dressing, frozen dinners, candy, breakfast cereal, granola bars, and canned soups.

Chapter 4: Eating Should Be Easy

Healthy eating should be easy. But go online, and what you'll see might make you question exactly what healthy eating is. In fact, the information overload might make you so overwhelmed that you pig out on junk food just to deal with the stress!

But eating healthy doesn't have to be stressful. The first step is to look at your current eating habits and then incorporate simple steps that will guide you on the path of eating real food.

Your Current Eating Habits

Reviewing and understanding your current eating habits can help you make the step to eating a balanced diet of real food. If you understand why you reach for certain foods, you can look at making changes. Perhaps you don't have a lot of time to cook a meal from scratch, or you like the taste of processed foods. Or maybe you follow someone on social media, and they extol the virtue of a certain diet. Or you may just not feel like taking the time to plan your weekly meals or make a grocery shopping list. Whatever the reason is, you must examine it.

One habit that is not conducive to healthy eating is getting takeout. Takeout food usually isn't the healthiest choice because it can be laden with salt and preservatives. Many times when you get takeout, the options are limited to white rice and things like white potatoes and bread.

Another thing you might do without realizing it is you pick up convenience or processed foods when you go grocery shopping. As you know, processed foods can be full of preservatives and are not the healthiest choice. But when you're pressed for time and want something to eat fast, convenience foods are tempting.

You could be eating certain foods because you're trying to lose weight, and you heard that a specific diet could help you lose weight fast. Or you are trying to lose weight by only drinking juice or fasting.

Consider keeping a food journal, or if you find that idea too stressful, you can jot down what you eat on a notepad on the kitchen counter. It doesn't have to be a big production. You just want to be able to reflect on what your current eating habits are.

Time to Make Simple Changes

Once you've examined your current eating habits, you can start looking at ways to make some simple changes.

The best way to control how healthy you eat is to cook your food at home. Want to try cooking food from scratch? Afraid that some recipes sound too complicated and that you don't have enough time? Remember that not all of your meals have to be fancy or complicated. Use the basic meal formula of protein + veggies and maybe a starch = dinner. This could look like grilled chicken and vegetables over brown rice. Or baked tofu and vegetables with quinoa.

If your weeks are usually busy with work and other activities, you can consider batch cooking on the weekend. Batch cooking is exactly what it sounds like. It means you prep and cook meals for a week or two. Then you store them in the fridge or freezer. Take one out every evening, reheat, and voila, dinner is served! Batch cooking is the best of both worlds. It allows you to enjoy healthy meals at home, and besides the time spent upfront when you do the prepping and initial cooking, it saves time during the week. It's almost as convenient as takeout but healthier.

If you want to try batch cooking, you can try it in small steps first. Think about what you might want to eat for three nights. Then make a grocery list, buy the ingredients, and set aside a couple of hours on a Saturday or Sunday afternoon or evening to do the prep and cooking. It might feel like you're spending a lot of time when you're preparing and cooking your meals, but during the week, when you take a meal out of the fridge and reheat it, you'll be amazed at how much extra time you have that evening.

You don't need to make new dishes every week. Keep it simple and repeat your meals so that you're not buying ingredients that you may not use again in the future. Plus, making the same or similar things means you will spend less time on preparing and cooking them in the future because you're familiar with how to do it.

Another simple tip is to not shop without a list. Shopping without a list means that you may be tempted to buy things that aren't the healthiest. Having a list makes it easier to stick with healthy options because you'll only need to go to the areas of the grocery store that have the things on your list. You should also not shop while you're hungry. When you're hungry, everything looks good, and the temptation to buy something junky is higher.

If you like to eat fish or chicken and tend to fry them, consider roasting, baking, broiling, slow-cooking, poaching, or stewing them instead. These different ways of cooking meat and fish don't produce the harmful compounds that are formed when you fry meat and fish, like polycyclic aromatic hydrocarbons, which have been linked to diseases like heart disease and cancer (Spritzler, 2020).

If you want to make one small step right away, you can plan to make one healthy meal per week. Again, it doesn't have to be complicated. Try it once and see for yourself! If it feels too overwhelming to make a healthy meal during the week, try making it on the weekend when you have a bit more time.

Next time you go grocery shopping, try picking up some healthier snacks so that you have healthy food readily available. It doesn't have to be a huge time constraint. Perhaps you buy a few carrots, cut them up, and put them in containers. Then, next time you're feeling peckish, you have some nice crunchy carrot sticks to snack on. Or buy raw, unsalted almonds in bulk and put some in different containers so that it's convenient for you just to grab a container either while you're on the go or while you're watching TV.

Try reading labels when you are out grocery shopping. You will get all the information you need with even a quick glance.

If you see words like 'modified' or 'hydrolyzed,' put the product back on the shelf. The same goes for labels with words that end in "ose" because that means sugars have been added to the product.

Make sure that you buy products whose labels have few ingredients. Healthy ingredients like whole grains and whole wheat should be listed in the top three on labels. And watch for salt content. Many companies put a lot of salt in their products to make them tastier (one reason why takeout food tastes so good).

If you get takeout, one little change you can make is to ask the restaurant to use brown rice instead of white or whole wheat pasta instead of white pasta in your meal. If they can't do that for you, is there a healthier alternative on their menu, or is there another restaurant that can make substitutes for you? The same goes if you're picking up a ready-made sandwich in the grocery store. Look for one with whole grain bread and real meat instead of processed meat slices.

When you're ordering takeout, many times, what you order as a main comes with a side. Instead of getting French fries or some type of cooked white potato on the side, consider having a side salad (with a vinaigrette dressing, not a creamy one) instead. If you're at a restaurant, think about ordering a salad as an appetizer so that you're guaranteed to get your vegetables in. And instead of ordering something fried, get it baked, steamed, grilled, or roasted. You can also ask for any sauce on the side, as typically, sauces are laden with salt and sugar.

Keeping healthy snacks where you can see them is another small thing you can do to eat healthier, real foods. Usually, when you're hungry, you eat the first thing you see. Keeping that container of almonds on a counter probably means that you'll snack on the almonds rather than something that is out of sight.

Another step to keep in mind is to count nutrients instead of calories. Counting calories can give you a deprivation mindset. It can also make you feel bad about yourself because you're comparing the calories you eat to a completely unsustainable and unreal goal.

Counting calories can be very misleading because it does not mean that you are eating healthier. If you set yourself up with a daily calorie limit, and you eat something with lots of empty calories (calories void of any nutritional value), you rob yourself of getting the nutrients you need. For example, if you treat yourself to a piece of chocolate cake, you may find that you don't have enough calories left in your allotted calorie intake for the day to eat something healthy like vegetables.

Calories are not all the same. Two different pieces of food may have the same number of calories but can provide your body with completely different nutritional value. On top of that, our bodies process calories from different foods in different ways so that the calories provide us with energy or make us lethargic. For example, a plate of whole grain pasta with lean protein will keep you more full than approximately two donuts with the same amount of calories.

Thinking only about calories means you are not considering the nutritional value of the food you are eating. For example, maybe you think that you shouldn't eat nuts because they have lots of calories. But think about how much energy you get from nuts and the nutritional value that nuts provide. Real, nutritious food will help you maintain stable blood sugar levels. It will also keep you full longer and reduce cravings.

Food that isn't nutritious will make your blood sugar levels spike, leading to feeling lethargic and possibly cranky. It also increases your cravings for more junk food.

Counting calories also robs you of the joys of eating because you can start to look at food as the enemy. You might think of it as something that will make you gain weight, instead of something that provides your body with nourishment and the energy to do your day-to-day activities. You might even find yourself becoming obsessed with counting calories.

Focusing on the quality of what you eat instead of the quantity can help if you find yourself thinking too much about calories. Thinking about how good the food is that you are putting in your body will lead you to continue eating healthier, quality food.

If you live with someone or have a friend or family member who is interested in trying to eat healthier, consider teaming up with them so that you are accountable to each other. You can take turns cooking a healthy meal and be there for each other if you give in to an unhealthy craving.

You don't have to make huge changes right now to start on the road towards healthier eating. Make one small step today or this week and see how you feel. The important thing is that you start.

Mindful Eating

Did you know that, on average, people make more than 200 decisions about food each day, and they're only aware of a small fraction of these decisions? (Harvard Health Publishing, 2016)

Most of the decisions you make about food each day are made by your unconscious mind. This can lead to mindless eating, which means you aren't thinking about the food you consume. Try to remember what you ate yesterday or even earlier today, and chances are you probably can't. That's probably because while you were eating, you were doing something else like watching TV, playing on your phone, working, or reading. You may have also eaten something really quickly before you moved on to your next activity.

Being mindful means focusing on the present moment. It means savoring our food while we eat it. It's also about being mindful when we shop, prepare, and cook our meals. That doesn't mean we have to eat five-star food at every meal, but it does mean enjoying our food at the moment.

One small thing you can do to incorporate mindful eating is to create a shopping list. Creating a list makes you think about what healthy meals you want to make during the week. It also helps you be more mindful about the types of things you put in your cart. This means you don't go into the grocery store and mindlessly wander the aisles putting things in your cart just because they look tasty. It also means you might spend less time wandering around your kitchen looking for something to snack on because you have already planned your meals and snacks.

Paying attention to your food also makes you appreciate what you have. If you pause for a moment before digging in and think about what's in front of you, you'll have an appreciation for what you're about to eat.

Think about all of the people who helped bring food to your table and feel grateful that you have the food you're about to eat. Thinking about where your food has come from can help you be more mindful. It helps you understand the connection between our natural world, farmers, all the other people involved in getting food to your table, and you. Being grateful for the healthy food you eat and how it makes you feel means you might find yourself eating unhealthy food less often.

When you're prepping your food, take your time. Put some of your favorite music on and really get into the food prep. You might be surprised at how much you enjoy chopping vegetables. Think of preparing your food as something to look forward to instead of a chore, and you might just appreciate your food a little bit more.

Also, try to use all of your senses when you are preparing, cooking, and eating your food. Look at the color, appreciate the texture and the smell of your food. Think about the sound that happens when you cut into a crispy red pepper. When you eat your food, think about all of the different flavors in it, even if it's just a simple dish.

Another tip for mindful eating is not to skip meals. Skipping meals means that you probably feel hungry often throughout the day. Feeling hungry usually means you will either reach for anything to alleviate your hunger, like junk food, or you'll stuff food in your mouth so quickly that you don't have time to think about it.

Try not to let yourself get too hungry during the day. This way, when mealtime comes, you can focus on eating your food slowly and not just on getting the food in you so fast so that you're no longer hungry.

Understanding your body and why you eat certain things can also help with mindful eating. If you're feeling stressed, bored, or emotional, you may tend to not focus so much on what you're putting in your body because you just want to feel better. This is where making that shopping list comes in handy. If you plan out what you want to have for meals and snacks for the week, you'll be able to better think of what healthy foods will bring you comfort if you find yourself stressed.

Taking smaller bites also helps you be more mindful. This goes back to not letting yourself get too hungry so that you're gulping your food. If you take smaller bites, you're able to better appreciate what you're eating. And remember to chew your food thoroughly. You want to taste your food before you swallow it!

This is a difficult one for many people but consider only eating when you're eating. What this means is when you sit down to eat, just eat. Don't text or play games on your phone. Don't scroll through the news. And maybe don't watch TV. Pay attention to what you're putting in your body.

Mindful eating doesn't have to be complicated. And remember that all you have is this present moment. You may as well enjoy it!

Eating Well for Life

You have read how important healthy, real food is to your body so that you can function at your best right now. But eating healthy now also makes a strong foundation for aging well in the future.

Eating some of the foods you have read about in this book is important for preventing inflammation and disease in the body. That becomes more important as you get older because being pain-free means that you will get to stay active for longer.

As we age, we lose muscle mass, and we sometimes also lose bone mass. Since we may not need as many calories as we age, it is important to make sure that the calories that we do eat are packed with nutrients.

A diet rich in real foods is important not only to our physical health as we age but also to our mental health. Alzheimer's disease is a disease associated with older adults, but it is not a normal part of aging. Eating anti-inflammatory foods can help fend off Alzheimer's. This is because inflammation can inhibit communication between brain cells and injure neurons (Melinda, 2019).

It is also important to keep your blood sugar levels balanced as you get older. Insulin resistance also contributed to injured neurons and inhibited communication between brain cells. Try to cut back on refined carbs and sugary foods.

Including vegetables, fruits, lean proteins, whole grains, olive oil, and fish will help your body and brain stay healthy into the future.

Treats and Snacks

What is life without the occasional treat? And snacks can play an important part in our daily lives and our social lives. When was the last time you had people over to watch a movie, and you didn't put out snacks?

There is a misconception that if you eat healthy, you never have a treat or don't snack. But there is a problem with depriving ourselves because if we think that we can't eat a certain food, we want it even more and may end up eating more of that food.

But the truth is that you can still snack and eat healthy at the same time. And there are a few hacks you can use to do both.

Lots of people want something salty and crunchy when they snack. The first things that come to mind are probably potato chips or French fries because they are quick, convenient, and so delicious. But they are high in bad fats and salt, which are not good for you.

What can you eat instead if you're craving a salty, crunchy snack? Try making kale chips. I know, I know but hear me out. It's simple to make. You have to cut up the kale, put it on a baking sheet and toss it with olive oil and salt. Bake until crispy, and voila, you have a crunchy, salty, healthier snack. You can also experiment with different flavors, like salt and vinegar, barbeque (use garlic powder, chili powder, dry mustard, brown sugar, and paprika), and cheeses (sprinkle with nutritional yeast). You can even make your kale chips and put them in individual baggies so that you have the option to grab and go anytime.

To replace french-fried potatoes, try making veggie fries instead. Put sweet potatoes, carrots, or parsnips in the oven and bake until crispy. When you take them out, you choose how much salt you put on them.

You can also make a healthy dip if you want, mixing garlic, Dijon mustard, or chipotle powder with some mayo. It's simple and delicious. You can also try using tzatziki as a dipping sauce. You can make your own with cucumber, yogurt, olive oil, lemon juice, garlic, fresh mint or dill, and a little salt.

If you are craving something sweet, there are healthy options for that too! Instead of ice cream, for example, you could try making your own frozen yogurt. Mix some of your favorite fruit and yogurt, put it in the freezer, and once it's frozen, you'll have a creamy, satisfying dessert. You can also try dipping a banana in dark chocolate and freezing it. If you're in the mood, you can make a big batch of frozen dessert so that it's on hand when you have a craving.

Try making energy bites with dates, nuts, and seeds instead of eating a donut. You won't have the crash from the excess sugar and the unhealthy carbs, and you'll probably have more energy to do the things you want to do.

You can also consider making a smoothie instead of getting a milkshake next time you crave a sweet drink. You can control the ingredients and make a delicious drink that contains nutrients and protein.

Instead of reaching for candy, think about dipping nuts in dark chocolate. And if you want something crunchy, freeze the nuts after dipping them in the chocolate. You can also dip fresh fruit in chocolate for a tasty treat.

You read earlier about replacing flour with black beans when making brownies. Well, there are many tips and tricks for substituting healthy ingredients if you plan on baking. For example, puree red beets until smooth and use them in place of oil in a cake recipe. They will add moisture to your cake, and you'll get your veggies too. Instead of using sugar in cakes and cookies, use monk fruit extract or stevia. They are natural sugar substitutes.

Chapter 5: You Can Do It!

As you read earlier, eating healthy should be easy and not stressful. Start small and see for yourself how much better you feel after adopting just one or two new habits.

Challenge Yourself

One fun way of trying out new habits is to challenge yourself and see how you do. Over the next couple of days or the next week, try one of the following. Or challenge yourself further by seeing how many things on the list you can do.

1. Grocery shopping: next time you go grocery shopping, only shop the perimeter of the store. That is where you will find real food, like produce, eggs, nuts, lean meats, and dairy. Avoid the center aisles because that is where the majority of the processed food is. You get bonus points if you plan your meals ahead of grocery shopping

and go prepared with a list. Extra bonus points for looking at the store's flyer ahead of time and planning your meals based on what's on sale!

2. Don't let yourself get too hungry during the day. As you read earlier, letting yourself get too hungry usually means that you will reach for convenience foods and/or not chew your food properly because you are eating too fast.

3. Start reading the labels on the food products you buy. If you're considering buying processed food, it should have less than five ingredients on the label that you can't pronounce. If it has more than that, ditch it.

4. Pay attention to how your body feels after you eat certain types of food. If you feel bloated, tired, lethargic, or your stomach hurts, consider it a sign that your body doesn't like the food you just ate. Listen to your body. It knows.

5. Add more colorful vegetables to your plate. You don't always have to eat a salad. You can switch it up and grill, bake, sear, or steam your vegetables. Or eat them raw and crunchy.

6. Drink more water than you normally would. If you don't like drinking plain water, you can add some natural flavor, like a lemon, orange, or cucumber slice. You can also put a few sprigs of mint in your water glass. Make drinking more water work for you!

7. Take deep breaths, clear your mind, go for a walk. Getting mindful for the rest of your life means you will be mindful about shopping for, prepping, cooking, and eating your food.

8. Buy local and seasonal produce where and when you can.

9. Don't count calories. Count nutrients. Instead of focusing on how many calories your food has, think about all of

the nutrients in it. All calories are not the same. It's the quality of the nutrients in the calories that counts and has the most impact on your health.

10. Remind yourself that home-cooked, real food is inexpensive, nutritious, and nourishing.

11. Don't beat yourself up if you eat a cookie, a slice of cake, or anything you didn't plan on eating. Be gentle with yourself. It's okay to enjoy a treat once in a while. But try not to eat processed, baked foods too often. Listen to how your body feels after you've eaten a treat and consider a healthier alternative.

You don't have to do this alone. Find a family member or friend to share this challenge with. Having an accountability buddy will make this challenge exciting. Having someone holding you accountable also means you will likely stay on track.

You've got this!

Chapter 6: Simple, Healthy Meal and Recipe Ideas

Starting on the road to healthier eating is exciting. You have read about how meal planning can help you eat healthier at home. Below you will find some simple ideas and recipes that are easy enough for a weekday or a weekend.

Breakfast

If you are in a rush and don't have time to eat breakfast at home, consider making boiled eggs the night before. Or you can chop up some fresh or dried fruit and put it in a container.

Fluffy Whole Wheat Banana Pancakes

Recipe from 100 Days of Real Food ("Fluffy Whole Wheat Banana Pancakes (Freeze the Leftovers!)", 2010)

Just because you're busy, it doesn't mean that you don't have time to eat healthy. Making these whole wheat banana pancakes means that you can eat them on the day that you make them and freeze the leftovers for another day. When you want to eat them again, take them out of the freezer, heat them, and breakfast is served. And you can make these even healthier by sprinkling some blueberries or chopped strawberries on top.

Servings: 4

Ingredients:

- 2 cups whole wheat flour
- 2 teaspoons baking powder
- 1 ½ teaspoons baking soda
- ½ teaspoon honey
- 2 eggs, lightly beaten
- 1 ¾ cups milk (you can substitute with non-dairy milk)
- 2 tablespoons butter (you can substitute with coconut oil)
- 2 bananas, mashed
- pure maple syrup, for serving

Instructions:

1. In a large bowl, mix the dry ingredients.
2. Make a hole in the center of the dry ingredients mixture and pour in the eggs, milk, honey, and two tablespoons of melted butter. Whisk together, but don't overmix.
3. Gently fold in the mashed bananas.
4. Heat a griddle or pan over medium-high heat. Melt enough butter to coat the pan. Add pancake batter with a measuring cup or a spoon.

5. When the pancakes have started to turn a golden brown color on the bottom, flip them over.
6. Serve with maple syrup and fruit on top or on the side.

Smoothie

Recipe from 100 Days of Real Food ("Recipe: Tasty Smoothies", 2010)

Smoothies are a great way to get breakfast on the go. And they help you get vegetables and fruit into your diet in a convenient way. Also, if you make enough, you can always put the leftovers in the fridge for the next day.

Servings: 2

Ingredients:

- 1.5 cups plain yogurt
- 1 cup berries (fresh or frozen)
- 2 bananas
- 2 tablespoons milk (or milk substitute)
- ½ cup spinach

Instructions:

1. Combine all ingredients in a blender. Pour into a cup and enjoy!

Whole Wheat Carrot Applesauce Muffins

Recipe from 100 Days of Real Food ("Whole Wheat Carrot Applesauce Muffins", 2013)

Homemade muffins are different from the muffins you can buy in stores. This is because you can control how much sugar and oil you put in them. You can make these muffins on the weekend and have a grab-and-go breakfast ready for the week. Even better if you pair one of these muffins with a banana!

Servings: 12

Ingredients:

- 1 ½ cups whole wheat flour
- 1 teaspoon baking soda
- 1 teaspoon ground cinnamon
- ½ teaspoon ground ginger
- ½ teaspoon salt
- ½ cup softened (not melted) butter
- ½ cup honey
- 1 egg
- 1 teaspoon pure vanilla extract
- 1 cup applesauce
- ¾ cup shredded carrots

Instructions:

1. Preheat the oven to 350°F. Place liners in your muffin tin.
2. Whisk the flour, baking soda, cinnamon, ginger, and salt in a medium bowl.

3. Mix the butter, honey, egg, and vanilla with an electric beater or whisk in a large bowl.
4. Turn the speed of the beater or whisk down and slowly add the flour mixture until the entire mixture is combined. Your batter should be thick.
5. Fold in the carrots and applesauce using a spatula.
6. Divide the batter between the muffin cups. Bake until muffins turn a golden brown or about 22 to 24 minutes.

Lunch

Lime-Cilantro Quinoa Salad

Recipe from 100 Days of Real Food ("Lime-Cilantro Quinoa Salad", 2011)

It can sometimes be easy to eat junk food at lunch because you may not find the time to make lunch at home and then find yourself buying fast food. But making a healthy lunch does not have to be complicated. You can make this quinoa salad as a side dish for dinner or make a big batch and store it in an air-tight container for lunches.

Servings: 6

Salad Ingredients:

- 3 cups cooked quinoa (equals 1 cup dry)
- ¾ cup dried fruit, like raisins or apricots
- ¼ pine nuts, toasted
- ¼ cilantro

- 1 bell pepper

Dressing ingredients:

- ¼ cup lime juice
- ¼ olive oil
- 1 teaspoon Dijon mustard
- 2 cloves garlic
- 1 pinch of salt

Instructions:

1. Mix all salad ingredients in a bowl.
2. Mix dressing ingredients in a separate bowl.
3. Pour the dressing over the salad, mix, and enjoy!

Vegetable Pancakes

Recipe from 100 Days of Real Food ("Recipe: Vegetable Pancakes", 2011)

These vegetable pancakes are very flexible in that you can use whatever vegetables you like and have in your house.

Servings: 2

Ingredients:

- 2 cups mixed vegetables, shredded (you could use sweet potatoes, carrots, squash, zucchini)
- 2 eggs
- 1 tablespoon whole wheat flour
- ¼ teaspoon salt
- olive oil, or coconut oil, for cooking
- optional garnishes: sour cream or applesauce

Instructions:

1. Combine shredded vegetables with flour, eggs, and salt.
2. Heat oil in a pan over medium heat. Make sure the pan is hot enough so that the pancakes heat in the middle as well as the outside.
3. Add pancake mixture to the pan. Cook until the bottom starts to brown, then flip.
4. Serve warm on their own or with sour cream or applesauce (or both!)

Whole Wheat Macaroni and Cheese

Recipe from 100 Days of Real Food ("Whole Wheat Macaroni and Cheese", 2010)

This whole wheat macaroni and cheese is just as easy as making the processed version from a box.

Servings: 4

Ingredients:

- 1 cup whole wheat macaroni, boiled according to instructions on the package
- 2 tablespoons butter
- 2 tablespoons whole wheat flour
- 1 cup milk
- 1 cup cheese, grated
- salt and pepper, to taste
- parmesan cheese, grated (optional)

Instructions:

1. Melt butter in a pan over medium heat.
2. Whisk in flour, then keep whisking for around one to two minutes until the mixture starts to darken.
3. Turn heat down and whisk in the milk. Turn the heat back up to medium and whisk until the mixture starts to get thick and all lumps are dissolved.
4. Stir in grated cheese.
5. Once cheese melts, stir in the cooked noodles.

If you are in a rush and don't have time to make something for lunch, you can grab a container of hummus and some pita to keep at work. It's even better if you can grab a cucumber to slice up and enjoy with your hummus and pita.

Dinner

Roasted (Summer) Vegetable Pasta

Recipe from 100 Days of Real Food ("Roasted {Summer} Vegetable Pasta", 2013)

Making a healthy, tasty dinner from scratch does not have to be complicated. If you're feeling tired on a weeknight, this pasta recipe will get you from the kitchen to the couch quickly!

Servings: 6

Ingredients:

- ½ lb whole wheat pasta, cooked according to instructions

- 1 eggplant, diced into 1 inch pieces
- 2 zucchinis, diced into 1 inch pieces
- 2 Roma tomatoes, diced into 1 inch pieces
- 2 cloves garlic
- ⅓ cup dry white wine
- 3 tablespoons olive oil
- 1 ½ tablespoon salt (add less if you're using tomato sauce with salt)
- 1 ¼ teaspoon thyme
- pepper, to taste
- 1 15-ounce can tomato sauce (preferably without salt)
- ¾ cup parmesan cheese, grated

Instructions:

1. Preheat the oven to 425 °F.
2. In a 13x9 casserole dish, combine the eggplant, zucchini, tomatoes, and garlic. Sprinkle wine, olive oil, and spices on top. Roast the vegetables for around 40 minutes, or until they are tender. Stir once halfway through cooking time.
3. Take the casserole dish out of the oven. Stir pasta and tomato sauce into vegetables. Top with parmesan cheese and put the casserole dish back into the oven for about five minutes, or until the cheese is melted.

Creamy Mushroom Vegetable Soup, With Barley

Recipe from 100 Days of Real Food ("Creamy Mushroom Vegetable Soup (with Barley)", 2014)

Making soup from scratch can be easy. Soup is a great way to batch cook. You can enjoy this recipe fresh or make it ahead of time for a convenient lunch or dinner.

Servings: 6

Ingredients:

- 4 tablespoons butter
- 4 shallots, minced
- 2 carrots, peeled and diced
- 1 stalk celery, diced
- 3 cloves garlic, minced
- 1 ½ pounds mushrooms, sliced
- ½ cup whole grain barley
- 4 cups vegetable or chicken broth
- ½ teaspoon salt and pepper to taste
- ¼ cup heavy cream

Instructions:

1. In a large soup pot, melt the butter over medium heat. Add the carrots, shallots, and celery and cook for about five to six minutes, until softened.
2. Add the garlic and mushrooms to the pot and cook for five more minutes.
3. Add the barley, broth, salt, and pepper and bring to a boil. Turn down the heat to a simmer and cook for about 30 to 40 minutes, until the barley is tender.
4. Stir in heavy cream and then serve.

Homemade Whole Wheat Pizza

Recipe from 100 Days of Real Food ("Homemade Whole Wheat Pizza", 2010)

Pizza night takes on a different meaning when you make the pizza yourself! Impress yourself and your family by making homemade, healthy pizza.

Servings: 4

Ingredients:

- 1 cup of water
- 2 tsp active dry yeast
- 2 tsp salt
- 2 tbsp olive oil
- 3 cups whole wheat flour
- tomato sauce (preferably without salt added)
- mozzarella cheese, grated
- oil spray
- Topping ideas:
- mushrooms
- mixed vegetables
- pesto
- goat cheese
- olives
- arugula
- sausage

Instructions:

1. Put the yeast into one cup of warm water. It should foam a little after a few minutes. Stir the olive oil and salt into the yeast mixture.
2. Mix the dough by hand or use a food processor.
3. You should end up with a dough ball that isn't too dry. If it is, add some warm water one teaspoon at a time. If your dough is too wet, add one teaspoon of flour at a time.
4. Knead the dough ball until it is smooth. Put the dough into a bag or bowl (with enough olive oil to coat the bag or bowl), cover, and put it in the fridge for at least one hour. You can also leave it overnight if you like.
5. When you are ready to make the pizza, preheat your oven to 500°F. Roll the dough until it's in a shape that you're happy with. Spray a baking sheet with cooking oil. Then put the dough on the baking sheet. Top the dough with tomato sauce and any other toppings that you like, including cheese.
6. Bake for around eight to ten minutes or until the pizza is a nice golden brown color.

Sweet Treats

Eating healthy doesn't mean you have to stop eating dessert as a treat once in a while. Try making one of these easy treats to satisfy your sweet tooth on a special occasion.

For regular days, try having fresh strawberries cut up in a bowl. You can drizzle them with a bit of melted dark chocolate if you want to jazz them up a little.

Or finish your meal with a small piece of dark chocolate. Dark chocolate has fiber and minerals, including magnesium, iron, copper, manganese, and potassium. It does have caffeine and sugar in it, of course, so enjoy in moderation.

Pumpkin Fluff Dessert Dip

Recipe from 100 Days of Real Food ("Pumpkin Fluff Dessert Dip", 2013)

Servings: 8

Ingredients:

- 1 cup heavy whipping cream
- ½ cup cream cheese
- 2 tablespoons maple syrup
- 1 teaspoon vanilla extract
- 1 teaspoon pumpkin pie spice
- 1 cup pumpkin puree
- Whole wheat crackers for dipping
- Apple slices for dipping

Instructions:

1. Mix heavy cream, cream cheese, syrup, vanilla, and pumpkin pie spice with an electric mixer. Combine until the mixture is smooth. Keep mixing for about one to two minutes, or until the mixture is thick.
2. Turn mixer speed to low and blend in pumpkin puree.
3. Serve with whole wheat crackers and apple slices.

Cinnamon Apple Crisp

Recipe from 100 Days of Real Food ("Cinnamon Apple Crisp (and Other Dinner Club Recipes!)", 2013)

Servings: 8

Filling ingredients:

- 2 large apples
- ¼ teaspoon cinnamon
- 1 tablespoon butter, melted
- 2 tablespoons honey

Crumble ingredients:

- ¾ cup rolled oats
- ½ cup whole wheat flour
- ½ cup walnuts, chopped
- 3 tablespoons butter, melted
- 2 tablespoons honey
- ¼ teaspoon salt

Instructions:

1. Preheat the oven to 375°F.
2. Slice the apples into 1-inch pieces.
3. In a bowl, mix apple pieces with cinnamon, honey, and butter.
4. Put apple mixture into a pie plate.
5. Combine crumble ingredients in a bowl.
6. Put crumble ingredients on top of the apple mixture.
7. Cover the pie plate and bake for 25 minutes. Remove the pie plate from the oven, remove the foil, place the pie

plate, bake in the oven and broil for two to three minutes or until the crumble topping is a light brown color.

Whole Wheat Crepes

Recipe from 100 Days of Real Food ("Whole Wheat Crepes (for Breakfast or Dessert!)", 2010)

Servings: 8

Ingredients:

- 3 eggs
- 1 cup whole wheat flour
- 1 cup milk
- ¾ cup honey
- 1 tablespoon honey
- 1 teaspoon vanilla extract
- ¼ teaspoon salt
- 1 tablespoon butter

Instructions:

1. Put all of the ingredients into a blender and mix. Let the ingredients stand for 15 minutes.
2. Melt butter in a pan over medium heat.
3. Pour a small amount of batter to thinly coat the pan. Swirl the batter around until the pan is coated.
4. Flip the crepe once it is brown on the bottom. Be careful not to tear it because it is very thin!
5. Cook for around one minute on the other side.
6. Serve with applesauce filling or pure maple syrup.

Conclusion

Good health starts with good food. Real, whole food can make a difference in how you feel and how your body functions. Listen to your body after you eat fast food. See what it tells you. Do you feel lethargic, tired, and maybe a bit grumpy? Now compare that to how you feel after eating a healthy meal. You'll probably find that you feel energetic, clear-headed, and ready to take on any challenge.

Eating healthy doesn't have to be complicated. And if you're cooking at home, your meals don't have to be fancy. Remember a basic formula of protein + veggies + maybe a starch and build your meals from there. It could be something as simple as grilled fish with a side salad or stir-fried tofu and vegetables over brown rice.

You can start your healthy-eating journey with baby steps. Maybe plan to make one healthy meal per week (try one of the recipes in this book!). Or try replacing your junky snacks with something healthier, like carrot sticks or almonds.

Being mindful about what you eat can also help you start your journey. Make a list of the ingredients you need to make your one healthy meal this week. And when you prep and cook, appreciate all of the different colors and sounds you see and hear as you chop and cook your vegetables. Take a moment of gratitude for all of the people who helped bring the food to your table. And when you eat, savor every bite.

Eating real food means that you will feel better now, and you will feel better later. A diet rich in healthy foods will help you stay healthy as you age because you will be able to keep inflammation and sugar spikes at bay. This is important for your physical and your mental health.

As you start on the road towards healthier eating, I encourage you to share this book with family and friends who might want to start their own journey to more healthy eating.

Did You Enjoy Reading Eat Well & Feel Great?

I want to say thank you for purchasing and reading this book!

If you liked reading this book and found some benefit in it, I'd love your support and hope that you could take a moment to post a review on Amazon. I'd love to hear from you, even if you have feedback, as it'll help me improve this book and others in the future.

I want to let you know that your review is very important to me and will help this book reach and impact more lives.

Thank you for your time and support!

References

American Heart Association. (2015). "Monounsaturated Fat." *Heart.org.* www.heart.org/en/healthy-living/healthy-eating/eat-smart/fats/monounsaturated-fats.

Bareuther, C. (2009). "Nutrition and Chronic Disease." *Todaysgeriatricmedicine.com,* www.todaysgeriatricmedicine.com/archive/010508pb.shtml.

Beck, J. (10 Mar. 2016). "More than Half of What Americans Eat Is 'Ultra-Processed.'" *The Atlantic.* www.theatlantic.com/health/archive/2016/03/more-than-half-of-what-americans-eat-is-ultra-processed/472791/.

Brinkworth, G. (9 Nov. 2009). "Long-Term Effects of a Very Low-Carbohydrate Diet and a Low-Fat Diet on Mood and Cognitive Function." *Archives of Internal Medicine,* vol. 169, no. 20. p. 1873, 10.1001/archinternmed.2009.329.

Chen, H., et al. (Sept. 2018). "Association between Dietary Carrot Intake and Breast Cancer." *Medicine,* vol. 97, no. 37. p. e12164, 10.1097/md.0000000000012164.

Cleveland Clinic (19 Mar. 2020). "7 Tips for Healthier Takeout." *Health Essentials from Cleveland Clinic.* health.clevelandclinic.org/7-tips-for-healthier-takeout/.

Cook, K. (8 June 2017). "7 Ways to Add Beans to Your Diet - Food & Nutrition Magazine." *Foodandnutrition.org,* foodandnutrition.org/blogs/student-scoop/7-ways-add-beans-diet/.

Domonoske, C. (2019). "NPR Choice Page." *Npr.org.* www.npr.org/sections/thetwo-way/2016/09/13/493739074/50-years-ago-sugar-industry-quietly-paid-scientists-to-point-blame-at-fat.

EatCleaner. (12 Jan 2017). "Why Clean Eating Doesn't Mean Deprivation". *EatCleaner.* eatcleaner.com/why-clean-eating-doesnt-mean-deprivation.

Elliott, B. (20 Jan. 2017). "7 Impressive Health Benefits of Yogurt." *Healthline.* www.healthline.com/nutrition/7-benefits-of-yogurt#TOC_TITLE_HDR_3.

Eske, J. (20 Nov. 2018). "Coconut Milk: Benefits, Nutrition, and Risks." *Medicalnewstoday.com.* www.medicalnewstoday.com/articles/323743#nutrition.

Ettinger, J. (1 Mar 2021). "New Research Finds Highly Processed Foods Are Actually Addictive." *The Beet.* thebeet.com/are-processed-foods-addictive-new-research-tells-why-you-cant-eat-just-one/.

Gearhardt, A., Hebebrand, J. (2 Feb. 2021). "The Concept of 'Food Addiction' Helps Inform the Understanding of Overeating and Obesity: YES." *The American Journal of Clinical Nutrition*, vol. 113, no. 2. pp. 263–267, pubmed.ncbi.nlm.nih.gov/33448279/, 10.1093/ajcn/nqaa343. Accessed 28 Apr. 2021.

Gunnars, K. (25 June 2018). "7 Proven Health Benefits of Dark Chocolate." *Healthline.* www.healthline.com/nutrition/7-health-benefits-dark-chocolate#TOC_TITLE_HDR_2.

Gunnars, K. (15 Nov. 2018). "Is Dairy Bad for You, or Good? The Milky, Cheesy Truth." Healthline, *Healthline Media.* www.healthline.com/nutrition/is-dairy-bad-or-good#nutrition.

Han, J., et al. (1 Feb. 2015). "The Effect of Glutathione S-Transferase M1 and T1 Polymorphisms on Blood Pressure, Blood Glucose, and Lipid Profiles Following the Supplementation of Kale (Brassica Oleracea Acephala) Juice in South Korean Subclinical Hypertensive Patients." *Nutrition Research and Practice*, vol. 9, no. 1. pp. 49–56, www.ncbi.nlm.nih.gov/pmc/articles/PMC4317480/, 10.4162/nrp.2015.9.1.49.

Harvard Health Publishing. (March 2011). "Meat or Beans: What Will You Have? Part Ll: Beans." *Harvard Health*, www.health.harvard.edu/staying-healthy/meat-or-beans-what-will-you-have-part-ll-beans

Harvard Health Publishing.(16 July 2015). "Carbohydrates — Good or Bad for You? - Harvard Health." *Harvard Health*, Harvard Health. www.health.harvard.edu/diet-and-weight-loss/carbohydrates--good-or-bad-for-you.

Harvard Health Publishing. (16 Jan. 2016). "8 Steps to Mindful Eating - Harvard Health." *Harvard Health*, Harvard Health. www.health.harvard.edu/staying-healthy/8-steps-to-mindful-eating.

Harvard Health Publishing. (Dec. 2018). "Legumes: A Quick and Easy Switch to Improve Your Diet - Harvard Health." *Harvard Health*, Harvard Health. www.health.harvard.edu/staying-healthy/legumes-a-quick-and-easy-switch-to-improve-your-diet.

Harvard Health Publishing. (11 Dec. 2019). "The Truth about Fats: The Good, the Bad, and the In-between - Harvard Health." *Harvard Health*, Harvard Health. www.health.harvard.edu/staying-healthy/the-truth-about-fats-bad-and-good.

Harvard School of Public Health. (20 Aug. 2018). "Vegetables and Fruits." *The Nutrition Source.* www.hsph.harvard.edu/nutritionsource/what-should-you-eat/vegetables-and-fruits/.

Harvard School of Public Health. (25 Sept. 2018). "Whole Grains." *The Nutrition Source.* www.hsph.harvard.edu/nutritionsource/what-should-you-eat/whole-grains/.

Harvard School of Public Health. (28 Oct. 2019). "Legumes and Pulses." *The Nutrition Source.* www.hsph.harvard.edu/nutritionsource/legumes-pulses/.

Harvard School of Public Health. (1 May 2020). "Nutrition and Immunity." *The Nutrition Source.* www.hsph.harvard.edu/nutritionsource/nutrition-and-immunity/.

Harvard School of Public Health. (19 Oct. 2020). "Dairy." *The Nutrition Source.* www.hsph.harvard.edu/nutritionsource/dairy/.

Hodgson, L. (10 Dec 2020)"15 Healthiest Vegetables: Nutrition and Health Benefits." *Medicalnewstoday.com.* www.medicalnewstoday.com/articles/323319.

Inspired Health. (14 June 2020). "What Are the Benefits of Batch Cooking?" *Inspired Health,* inspiredhealth.co.uk/ blogs/wellness/what-are-the-benefits-of-batch-cooking#:~:text=One%20of%20the%20biggest%20benefits.

Jacobs, D., et al. (June 2007). "whole Grain Consumption Is Associated with a Reduced Risk of Noncardiovascular, Noncancer Death Attributed to Inflammatory Diseases in the Iowa Women's Health Study." *The American Journal of Clinical Nutrition,* vol. 85, no. 6. pp. 1606–1614, 10.1093/ajcn/85.6.1606.

Joseph, M. (23 Feb 2021)."56 Different Types of Vegetables and Their Nutrition Profiles." *Nutrition Advance,* www.nutritionadvance.com/healthy-foods/types-of-vegetables/#tab-con-1.

Leake, L. (1 Apr. 2010). "Homemade whole Wheat Pizza." *100 Days of Real Food.* www.100daysofrealfood.com/ recipe_homemade_whole_wheat_pizza/.

Leake, L. (21 Apr. 2010). "Fluffy whole Wheat Banana Pancakes (Freeze the Leftovers!)." *100 Days of Real Food.* www.100daysofrealfood.com/recipe-whole-wheat-banana-pancakes-freeze-the-leftovers/.

Leake, L. (17 May 2010). "Recipe: Tasty Smoothies." *100 Days of Real Food.* www.100daysofrealfood.com/recipe-tasty-smoothies/.

Leake, L. (16 Aug. 2010). "whole Wheat Crepes (for Breakfast or Dessert!)." *100 Days of Real Food.* www.100daysofrealfood.com/recipe-crepes-for-breakfast-or-dessert/.

Leake, L. (31 Dec. 2010). "whole Wheat Macaroni and Cheese." *100 Days of Real Food.* www.100daysofrealfood.com/recipe-whole-wheat-macaroni-and-cheese/.

Leake, L. (14 June 2011). "Lime-Cilantro Quinoa Salad." *100 Days of Real Food.* www.100daysofrealfood.com/recipe-lime-cilantro-quinoa-salad/.

Leake, L. (26 Aug. 2011). "Real Food Tips: 22 On-The-Go Breakfast Ideas." *100 Days of Real Food.* www.100daysofrealfood.com/real-food-tips-22-on-the-go-breakfast-ideas/.

Leake, L. (12 Sept. 2011). "Recipe: Vegetable Pancakes." *100 Days of Real Food.* www.100daysofrealfood.com/recipe-vegetable-pancakes/.

Leake, L. (18 July 2013). "Roasted {Summer} Vegetable Pasta." *100 Days of Real Food.* www.100daysofrealfood.com/recipe-roasted-summer-vegetable-pasta/.

Leake, L. (25 Oct. 2013). "whole Wheat Carrot Applesauce Muffins." *100 Days of Real Food.* www.100daysofrealfood.com/recipe-whole-wheat-carrot-applesauce-muffins/.

Leake, L. (14 Nov. 2013). "Pumpkin Fluff Dessert Dip." *100 Days of Real Food.* www.100daysofrealfood.com/recipe-pumpkin-fluff-dessert-dip/.

Leake, L. (19 Nov. 2013). "Cinnamon Apple Crisp (and Other Dinner Club Recipes!)." *100 Days of Real Food.* www.100daysofrealfood.com/cinnamon-apple-crisp-recipedinner-club/.

Leake, L. (13 Feb. 2014). "Creamy Mushroom Vegetable Soup (with Barley)." 100 Days of Real Food. www.100daysofrealfood.com/recipe-creamy-mushroom-vegetable-soup-barley/.

Limdico, Patrick. (22 May 2020). "57 Critical Fast Food Industry Statistics and Trends (2020 Update)." *Foodtruckempire.com.* foodtruckempire.com/news/fast-food-statistics/.

Lisa, A. (17 Jan 2020). "50 Ways Food Has Changed in the Last 50 Years." *Stacker,* stacker.com/stories/2500/50-ways-food-has-changed-last-50-years.

Martínez Steele, E., et al. (3, Jan. 2016). "Ultra-Processed Foods and Added Sugars in the US Diet: Evidence from a Nationally Representative Cross-Sectional Study." *BMJ Open,* vol. 6, no. p. e009892, bmjopen.bmj.com/content/6/3/e009892, 10.1136/bmjopen-2015-009892.

Marventano, S., et al. (31 Aug. 2016). "Legume Consumption and CVD Risk: A Systematic Review and Meta-Analysis." *Public Health Nutrition,* vol. 20, no. 2. pp. 245–254, www.cambridge.org/core/services/aop-cambridge-core/content/view/F2200011FB96DD7598704A4839CDC46A/S1368980016002299a.pdf/legume_consumption_and_cvd_risk_a_systematic_revi ew_and_metaanalysis.pdf, 10.1017/s1368980016002299.

Migala, J. (20 Feb 2020). "Here's Why a Sugar Crash Slows You down — and How to Boost Your Energy." *LIVESTRONG.COM*, www.livestrong.com/article/461919-sleepy-after-eating-sweets/.

Miller, S. (23 Jan 2017). "11 Ways Processed Food Is Different from Real Food." *Livescience.com*, www.livescience.com/57581-processed-food-differences.html.

National Cancer Institute. (2010). "Cruciferous Vegetables and Cancer Prevention." *National Cancer Institute, Cancer.gov.* www.cancer.gov/about-cancer/causes-prevention/risk/diet/cruciferous-vegetables-fact-sheet.

National Institutes of Health. (2016). "Office of Dietary Supplements - Vitamin C." *Nih.gov.* ods.od.nih.gov/factsheets/VitaminC-HealthProfessional/.

NutritionData. (2018). "Peppers, Sweet, Red, Raw Nutrition Facts & Calories." *Nutritiondata.self.com*, nutritiondata.self.com/facts/vegetables-and-vegetable-products/2896/2.

O'Connor, A. (18 Feb. 2021). "Unhealthy Foods Aren't Just Bad for You, They May Also Be Addictive." *The New York Times.* www.nytimes.com/2021/02/18/well/eat/food-addiction-fat.html?auth=-google1tap.

Pendick, D. (18 June 2015). "How Much Protein Do You Need Every Day?" Harvard *Health Blog.*

www.health.harvard.edu/blog/how-much-protein-do-you-need-every-day-201506188096#:~:text=The%20Recommended%20Dietary%20Allowance%20(RDA.

Petre, A. (11 Apr. 2019). "13 Science-Backed Tips to Stop Mindless Eating." Healthline, *Healthline Media*. www.healthline.com/nutrition/13-tips-to-stop-mindless-eating.

Robinson, L., et al. (2019). "HelpGuide.org." *HelpGuide.org*. www.helpguide.org/articles/healthy-eating/choosing-healthy-protein.htm.

Safety Hunters. (22 Feb. 2019). "Why Do We Need Food to Survive: A Detailed Answer." *Safety Hunters*. safetyhunters.com/why-do-we-need-food-to-survive-a-detailed-answer/.

Selhub, E. (5 Apr. 2018). "Nutritional Psychiatry: Your Brain on Food - Harvard Health Blog." *Harvard Health Blog*, Harvard Health Publishing. www.health.harvard.edu/blog/nutritional-psychiatry-your-brain-on-food-201511168626.

Services, PearlPoint Nutrition. (27 June 2012). "REAL Food, What's the Difference?" *PearlPoint Nutrition Services®*. pearlpoint.org/real-food-whats-difference/.

Smith, M. , et al. (28 Mar. 2019). "HelpGuide.org." *HelpGuide.org*. www.helpguide.org/articles/alzheimers-dementia-aging/preventing-alzheimers-disease.htm.

Spritzler, F. (11 Aug 2020). "21 Reasons to Eat Real Food." *Healthline.* www.healthline.com/nutrition/21-reasons-to-eat-real-food#TOC_TITLE_HDR_4.

Steen, J. (11 Oct. 2016). "Why You Should Stop Counting Calories (and Count Nutrients Instead)." *Huffington Post.* www.huffingtonpost.com.au/2016/10/11/why-you-should-stop-counting-calories-and-count-nutrients-inste_a_21475199/. Accessed 28 Apr. 2021.

Strang, S., et al. (12 June 2017). "Impact of Nutrition on Social Decision Making." *Proceedings of the National Academy of Sciences*, vol. 114, no. 25. pp. 6510–6514, www.pnas.org/content/114/25/6510.abstract, 10.1073/pnas.1620245114.

Szalay, J. (15 July 2017). "What Are Carbohydrates?" *Live Science.* www.livescience.com/51976-carbohydrates.html.

Taggart, S. (16 Oct. 2019). "How Food Has Changed in the Past 50 Years". *Eco18.* Collectively Green. eco18.com/how-food-has-changed-in-the-past-50-years/.

U.S. Department of Agriculture. (n.d.) "Fruits | MyPlate." *Myplate.gov*, www.myplate.gov/eat-healthy/fruits.

Warwick, K. (16 Jan 2020). "9 Health Benefits of Beans." *Medicalnewstoday.com*, www.medicalnewstoday.com/articles/320192#benefits.

Willard, C. (17 Jan. 2019). "6 Ways to Practice Mindful Eating - Mindful." *Mindful.* www.mindful.org/6-ways-practice-mindful-eating/.

World Health Organisation. (29 Apr. 2020). "Healthy Diet." *Who.int*, World Health Organization: WHO. www.who.int/news-room/fact-sheets/detail/healthy-diet.

Van Edwards, V. (1 June 2019). "Why Do We Eat? 10 Amazing Science Facts behind Our Eating Habits." *Science of People.* www.scienceofpeople.com/why-we-eat/#:~:text=We%20eat%20because%20we%20are.

Vespa, J. (24 Oct 2016). "The Importance of Protein in a Balanced Diet." *Cooking Light,* www.cookinglight.com/eating-smart/nutrition-101/what-is-the-purpose-of-protein.

Yamamoto-Taylor, B. (30 May 2018). "15 Healthy Alternatives to Junk…" *Cook Smarts,* Cook Smarts. www.cooksmarts.com/articles/15-healthy-alternatives-to-junk-food/.

Printed in Great Britain
by Amazon

16184060R00058